THIRD EYE AWAKENING

II

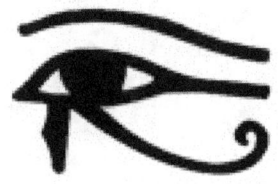

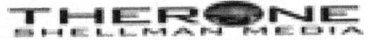

THERONE SHELLMAN

Order Therone Shellman Books At
www.amazon.com/author/theroneshellman

Authors Note

Talks become heated when, the health debate
comes up regarding, whether a meat, vegetarian,
or 100% plant based diet, is the best for humans.
It's obvious, since this book, leans more toward the
vegetarian and vegan lifestyle, what side I lean
towards. Nevertheless, the goal of the book is for
everyone to obtain optimal health. So, let's go.
Plus, according to the (ADA) American Dietetic
Association, throughout history most of the human
population has lived on a non meat diet.

ISBN-978-1540307750

ISBN-1540307751

Published by Therone Shellman Media
Edited by BlackInk
Proofread: Therone Shellman Media

www.amazon.com/author/theroneshellman
www.theronesmedia.com
www.facebook.com/author/theroneshellman
www.twitter.com/TheroneSMedia
www.instagram.com/theroneshellmanmedia

This book is dedicated to all the humans, who are seeking a better way to think, live, and eat. Hopefully, we can become more thoughtful, and concerned with the welfare of all life forms in the, universe.

CONTENTS

INTRODUCTION

So much emphasis is placed on spiritual and mental health, without making the connection with physical health. The holistic health of a human if it's to be practiced or administered right is to incorporate a daily regimen, which includes thoughts and actions, which concern the spiritual, mental and physical health, of the individual.

In 1990, I became a vegetarian after becoming sick due to eating, spaghetti and meatballs. Up until this point it was my favorite meal. For some reason, I never been too thrilled about the practice of eating meat, and even as a teen felt it wasn't the best food to consume health wise. A little while later, I would go on to read, How to Eat to Live by Elijah Muhammad, and then works by the world renowned Dr. Andrew Weil.

The purpose, of this work is to encourage people to begin to live a healthier lifestyle, or to further enlighten, those on the path to greater enlightenment into the health of the, whole Self.

The Mind and Body operate as one. In Eastern medicine, to treat a physical ailment, the spiritual and mental Self is dealt with. As it's believed all sickness, has its root in the mind. In the Western world, the mind, body, and spirit are treated as different entities, in regards to the practice of health. One is given medication, which purely serves as a remedy, not a cure. It solves the symptoms, not the cause of the sickness. Therefore, one never learns to practice healthy living, and a lifestyle to avoid such, sickness again. More times than not, once again they're back on medication, which only provides a remedy to such symptoms. It's no wonder why the pharmaceutical industry, is a trillion dollar industry.

Third Eye Awakening II is designed to enlighten people on how to be active participants in their body's health. There's a popular saying, which applies here very well. "What you don't use, you lose." The saying definitely applies to the health of the physical body. The less one is active, the less their metabolism, body muscles, and organs operate. The less one knows about how the mind, body and spirit operate as one. The more one tends to not pay attention to the needs of the whole Self. It's like driving a car consistently without getting a tune up.

Anyone can learn from and apply the principles to their life. But the drive to write this book is meant to educate the African American population, and diaspora in regards to physical health. As a result of slavery, they've taken on living and eating habits, which are detrimental to their health. Third Eye Awakening primarily deals with the origins of spirituality from a historical perspective. The work does take the time to highlight how the major religions borrowed from African spiritual and social systems. This is in itSelf, a very important part of human history, missing from most Western historical and spiritual works. Part II is to empower the physical Self. Again, it must be stressed that anyone can learn from the points mentioned in the book. Health is universal human need, and it applies to all.

Humans are taught to chase the riches of this world, at the expense of their health. The fun, enjoyment, and pleasures, are to be explored by destroying Self, as a result of drugs, alcohol, and consuming poisonous foods. For most, the glitter and gold of the world, has more value, than Self.

THIRD EYE

AWAKENING

II

"In this lifetime, you'll only have one body. How you take care of it, will determine, how, and to what ability, you'll be able to navigate this world."

Let's Get Healthy!

HEALTH

The body is your temple

The body is the house of the human spirit, and Intelligence of the universe. Intelligence is expressed and understood by humans through the thinking and actions of humanity as a result of the spirit, mind, and body. Our lifespan, in each lifetime is primarily dependent upon such factors as the quality of thought, and action, as well as how well we maintain our physical compositions.

The human body is like a car. In fact it's needier than a car in regards to care. A car needs its oil changed regularly, a tune up, tires changed, and overall regular maintenance. If one beats their car up, by not having maintenance done, and over accelerating the engine and driving too fast, or bumping and crashing into objects. The car will not be in operation for long. In other words, you'll need a replacement, sooner or later. The unfortunate thing about the human body is that there is no replacement; at least in this lifespan. You cannot go on, and purchase another body. The one you have is it. If you take care of it, or abuse it. The fact remains that you'll not have access to another one.

In order to navigate this world, conquer the environment, as well as cooperate with the elements in it. We must work with our bodies to create, and express the dreams of the universe, through creating, and our labor. The human body consists of 270 bones, 14 systems, but the major systems of the body are the muscular system, circulatory system, digestive system, respiratory system, excretory system, and skeletal system. The human body has the ability to heal itSelf, in accordance with healthy thought, diet and physical regimen. Just as well as ill, negative thoughts have the ability to bring the body sickness.

"I've always been a firm believer in taking care of my body since teen hood. For some reason I rationalized at a young age, that I was going to need my body for my whole life. How well, I take care of it, is going to have a lot to do with, it's condition when I reach an old age. Things happen like, freak accidents, car accidents, etc. But for the most part I've never, and wouldn't ever take the responsibility of taking care of myself away from Self. I'm responsible for my own health, and I have to take every precaution to ensure, I'm in the best shape possible. Being an author, and getting around reminds me daily, of the need to take care of myself, and the realization that had I not started taking my health seriously young, I possibly wouldn't be able to get around like I do. The majority of my book sales come from meeting people face to face, doing signings, and travelling. I'm on my feet a lot. So, I know firsthand, how one's physical health also has a lot to do with their ability to earn."

The human body is the product of DNA and genetic history

According to new biological studies Africans who have had no interbreeding with other groups, such as Caucasians, Asians, Indians are the true Homosapiens; 100% humans. These people (Africans) migrated up into Europe, and encountered the Neanderthal species (which are the ancestors of the Caucasian race) and they interbred. One might state, "What difference does this make?" Well, the book is about physical health, food diet practices, and its affects physically, mentally and spiritually. The history of these different species, in many ways explains our eating habits today. Just because most of the population consumes meat, doesn't mean it has always been so, or that it's the correct eating and health choice for humans.

Each group of people scattered around the globe have developed habits, which has become a part of their DNA and genetic history. Their spiritual practices, eating habits, living lifestyle, and physical activities, have all become lodged within their DNA; which is equivalent to a computer chip. Within the DNA is all of a humans recorded history; the triumphs and failures. It's the same with all beings. The development of the groups physical stature. The result of the environment they've mainly resided in, their activities and the species they evolved from; hence the, African, Caucasians, Asians, Indians, etc.

When one comes from an athletic and physically active family the males tend to be born with the ability to develop muscular bodies, easier than someone who may come from a family, who for many generations primarily weren't athletic, or utilized their bodies to work, lift, etc.

"From having associates who breed dogs, I've always been aware of bloodlines, and how many traits are hereditary, and passed down from generation to generation. This isn't just limited to the physical composition, but mentalities also play a part, and are affected by bloodline. A perfect example, which can be used is how generations of people who experience oppression, can actually possess symptoms similar to PTSD. These symptoms are passed down to the next generation, just like any other trait. I've been studying social studies, and social inequalities. It's helped me to realize that human behavior, and society, has a lot to do with genetic history, within groups, and individuals. How we look, and think, has everything to do with ancestry, and generational world experience."

The food one consumes, also affects their mental health

More and more health research is showing that the food one consumes does have an effect on one's mood, and mental health. The documentary 'Super Size Me' takes you through the experience of a man, who only consumes McDonald's food 3 times a day, for 30 days. Everything he consumes, even water is bought from McDonald's. He doesn't exercise, and he tries his best to restrict physical activity. As a result of eating the food, he gains weight, develops high cholesterol, and high blood pressure, by the middle of the month.

The website webmd.com in their article "Can What You Eat Affect Your Mental Health?" states via psychiatrist Drew Ramsey, MD an assistant clinical professor at Columbia University, "The risk of depression increases about 80% when you compare teens with the lowest quality diet, or what we call the Western diet, to those who eat a higher-quality, whole-foods diet. The risk of attention-deficit disorder (ADD) doubles."

"I've been a vegetarian since 1990, and am slowly making the transition to vegan. After eating spaghetti and meatballs, and getting very sick I decided that eating beef was going to end. At the time I had ceased consuming pork for about two years. Nevertheless, I do from personal experience understand the relationship of food diet, and mental health. When I eat a plate of spaghetti and sauce, I tend to just want to relax. Whereas, if I eat some peanut butter sandwiches, I feel totally different and am more alert and energized. Throughout the day to get a little boost, I usually eat (fruit trail mix) some peanuts, raisins, dried banana chips, dried apricot. Or some honey roasted peanuts."

Eating the wrong foods can cause one to gain weight, and become obese. This contributes in many cases to one developing negative thoughts about themselves.

"My whole life, I've been physically active, and in pretty good shape. It's helped me to feel good about myself, and I've always loathed the idea of becoming obese. I place health above having money, honestly. I cannot grasp how people will take care of a car, house, motorcycle, or put countless hours into a job weekly. Yet, give no time to exercise, or little thought to food nutrition. One is obviously, saying to themselves, they care about these things, more than they care about themselves."

We have to change our whole perception about health

Out of the business, civic and spiritual sectors of the Black community, the only ones who have consistently emphasized physical health, along with spiritual and mental throughout the decades is the Nation of Islam. The Jehovah Witnesses do publish pamphlets which cover health issues. Most Religious sectors will stress spirituality, yet will overlook physical health completely, and tend to speak little of mental health. Christian pastors, often make halfhearted attempts at speaking to their congregations about physical health. This is possibly due to the fact that many denominations follow the New Testament, as opposed to the King James Version. Leviticus Chapter 11 explicitly covers what animals, bird, and sea creatures not to eat. Many Christians eat the pig, although they're advised not to eat it. All creatures in the sea and rivers which don't have fins or scales are not to be eaten; shrimp, shell fish, etc. The Qur'an and Bible speak intimately about health in mind, spirit and body. Both texts provide instruction, as to the proper foods to eat. Yet, most pastors and imams see their institutions members are obese, and in physical distress. Their cups are always half empty, or full. It doesn't matter, half full, or half empty. It's just word, and mind games, because in physical reality it amounts to the same.

"I started reading books on African American history young. So I learned of the Tuskegee Syphilis Experiment. Where African American men were used as test dummies to see the effects on one's health when one isn't treated for the disease. I've also read about many experiments also done on Black prisoners. Today, it's a known practice that many doctors receive kickbacks from drug companies, to promote their drugs. Let's just say, all this knowledge and insight, has caused me to have distrust for doctors and the American health system in general. So, I've learned to take care of myself."

According to Wikipedia:

The **Tuskegee Study of Untreated Syphilis in the Negro Male**, also known as the **Tuskegee Syphilis Study** or **Tuskegee Syphilis Experiment** (/tʌsˈkiːɡiː/ _tus-**KEE**-ghee_) was an infamous clinical study conducted between 1932 and 1972 by the U.S. Public Health Service studying the natural progression of untreated syphilis in rural African-American men in Alabama under the guise of receiving free health care from the United States government.

The Truth about consuming Meats

The (ADA) American Dietetic Association notes that "most of mankind for most of human history has lived on vegetarian or near-vegetarian diets."

The human body isn't designed to digest and ingest meat. Carnivores, have claws, perspire through their tongue, and possess sharp front teeth with no flat molars for grinding, and an intestinal tract, which is only three times their body length so that meat passes through the digestive system quickly. This, is all the opposite for humans who possess no claws, perspire through their skin pores, have no sharp teeth, possess stomach acid that is 20 times weaker than carnivores, alkaline saliva, and an intestinal tract 10 to 20 times their body length.

The question about why humans consume meat can possibly be found in the history of the species. The origin of Homosapiens (humans) started in Africa. Africans migrated to different parts of the planet. When they arrived in Europe, they encountered the Neanderthals, which are the ancestors of the European race. They also encountered other species. Of course they interbred with these species, who were less evolved in Intelligence than Homosapiens, who already had thriving civilizations in Africa. None of these species, possessed the knowledge of civilization, and were living savage like until Africans found them.

Needless to say they weren't farming, etc. Their diet was flesh, primarily.

Naturally carnivores, eat meat raw. It can be assumed that the Neanderthals, and other species consumed raw flesh. Somewhere along the lines of Europe developing civilizations, and the Neanderthals and other species being overcome by the Homosapiens (Africans) those who still maintained a flesh diet, started cooking the meat. This alone, expresses the genetic code of consciousness within humans, expressing that it's not natural to consume meat. Naturally carnivores eat their meat raw.

Food is one form of fuel to the body

Your physical composition is your temple, and just like a car needs proper maintenance, so does your body. In fact one's body is needier. Most of your capabilities will be partly due to how you take care of your physical composition.

"When I look back upon my personal experiences, in relation to physical health and nutrition, three individuals come to mind, the Honorable Elijah Muhammad, Dr. Andrew Weil, and the late Dr. Sebi.

As a teen I became a member of the Nation of Gods & Earths (5% Percent Nation.) From day one I was instructed into the practice of fasting. For three days I ate only fruit, drank water, and was given some lessons to begin studying. I truly believe in the Honorable Elijah Muhammad's system of combining fasting with a proper diet, to maintain health. A year or so later I would become a vegetarian. This was over 25 years ago, and to this day I hold dear to the system. Right now, I'm embarking on the journey into Veganism. Little by little, because I still crave cheese."

You attract that which you're calling out to. About a year after reading How to Eat to Live, I stumbled upon a book by Dr. Andrew Weil. I cannot remember the first title I read by him, as it was so long ago. But I do remember the book was based upon naturopathic health, and food nutrition. I recall reading about different food diets, which in some cases have been helpful in curing cancer, and other illnesses. What intrigued me most about his books is the fact that he's travelled around the globe to meet indigenous people, and find their natural earthly cures to various ailments.

In 2010 I was set up with my books, and selling some other products. A gentleman approached me, and we began to speak about HIV, and he started to talk about Dr. Sebi and his work. He mentioned that the doctor found, an all natural herbal cure to the virus, and he was actually teaching that through a proper alkaline based diet one can avoid many ailments, and diseases, as well as cure them. Ever since becoming a vegetarian, I became a quick believer in the benefits, of a healthy diet. So I snatched up the paperwork he had, and I also took the time to listen to many of the internet phone talks Dr. Sebi, and those of his supporters administered. Very interesting, was my thoughts out the gate. I learned so much about diet, and biochemically engineered food through his work. Many of the vegetables, nuts, grains, herbs, most people consume, are really useless, in the health sense, as his research explains. When one thinks of eating healthy, one has to acknowledge that it's way more than just eating vegetables, and fruit. It's important to do research, because some vegetables and fruit possess very poor nutritional value. Below, I've included some info on proper nutrition according to Dr. Sebi's diet.

Vegetables

Amaranth greens (a type of spinach)
Avocado
Bell Peppers
Chayote (Mexican Squash)
Cucumber
Dandelion greens
Garbanzo beans
Green banana
Izote- cactus flower-cactus leaf

Kale
Lettuce (all except Iceberg)
Mushrooms (all except Shitake)
Nopales (Mexican Cactus)
Okra
Olives
Onions
Greens
Sea Vegetables (wakame, dulse, arame, hijiki, nori)
Squash
Tomato (cherry and plum)
Turnip greens
Zucchini
Watercress
Purslane (Verdolaga)

Fruits

"No canned or seedless fruits"

Apples
Bananas (the smallest one or the mid size, original banana)
Berries (no cranberries)
Cantaloupe
Cherries
Currants
Dates
Figs
Grapes (seeded)
Limes (key limes with seeds)
Mango
Melons (seeded)

Orange (Seville or sour preferred)
Papayas
Peaches
Pear
Plums
Prickly Pear (Cactus Fruit)
Prunes
Raisins (seeded)
Soft Jelly Coconuts
Soursops (Latin or West Indian markets)
Tamarind

Herbal Teas

Allspice
Anise
Burdock
Chamomile
Elderberry
Fennel
Ginger
Raspberry
Tila

Spices and Seasonings

Mild Flavors

Basil
Bay leaf
Cloves

Dill
Oregano
Parsley
Savory
Sweet Basil

Pungent and Spicy Flavors

Achiote
Cayenne
Cilantro
Habanero
Sage

Salty Flavors

Pure Sea Salt
Powdered Granulated Seaweed (Kelp, Dulce, Nori)

Sweet Flavors

100% Pure Agave Syrup
Date Sugar

Grains

Amaranth
Fonio
Kamut
Quinoa

Rye
Spelt
Tef
Wild Rice

Nuts and Seeds (includes Nut and Seed Butters)

Hemp Seed
Raw Sesame Seeds
Raw Sesame Tahini Butter
Walnuts
Brazil Nuts
Pine Nuts

Oils

Olive Oil (Do not cook)
Coconut Oil (Do not cook)
Grapeseed Oil
Sesame Oil
Hempseed Oil
Avocado Oil

Learn more at DrSebisCellFood.com
May you continue to live his legacy.

I must add, that Dr. Sebi dedicated his life mission to re-educate the African diaspora and Indigenous people, about health and dietary food practices. He understood that due to the Transatlantic slave trade to the America's, the invasion of Australia by Europeans, the enslavement of people of African descent, Indians and

Indigenous people upon the continents of the Western hemisphere, and the islands of the West Indies (Puerto Rico, Cuba, Jamaica, Haiti, Barbados, Unites States Virgin Islands), the people were colonized mentally and physically. All were stripped of their cultures, and way of life.

Dr. Sebi as a naturopathic practitioner believed that the human body could cure it's itSelf. With an alkaline diet, one would be able to rid their body of toxins, and disease.

One's diet also is a reflection on their views of life

Humans, are mammals, but quite more evolved in Intelligence than other species of mammals. Yet, the fact remains that humans, are mammals. The earth exists, as a home, and place to provide all mammals and all other creatures of flesh with all of their necessities. How can humans claim to be so intelligent and the leaders of all of life on this planet, when they're consuming other animals, and creatures of flesh? It doesn't make much sense does it? The very definition of civilization embodies order, and cooperation. The Homosapien (human) species, beat out the Neanderthals, and other species, because they were more evolved in Intelligence. Had they been on the same wild, and uncivilized thinking level of all the other species, it's quite possible the human species, may of went the way of the Neanderthals.

Humans, are envisioning the dream of the universe within, and expressing it out, through creation. Therefore, they have the ability to become one with the dream. This answers the question as to if, man is God. Or why do the scriptures state, that humans are gods.

What one consumes mentally, and physically, feeds the spirit. The spirit is ones eternal Self. Therefore, what one chooses to eat, is a direct reflection, on their views of, Self.

All of life is connected to one universal power

The same Intelligence, which manifested the Universe(s), exists within all plains of energy, and creations (manifestations.) This also means you, and I. Yes, you, I will state it again. So, while you're looking here and there for a savior. Know that you're connected to an omnificent force, and power.

Let's look at it like this. In your house there's a main electricity circuit box. Within the box, is switches which control all of the electrical outlets in the home, by sections. Each electrical outlet possesses its own potential, and level of power. This is the same with all things in existence. Minerals, plants, animals, and humans, all possess the potential rise to certain levels of intelligence. Within each group, there are also levels of intelligence and potential.

Food nutrition just doesn't affect you. It also affects your future generations.

It's obvious that during the slave trade to the America's, the slaves weren't treated well physically. They were also taught how to eat the wrong foods. In turn, they learned to cook the parts of the animals that the plantation owners didn't eat themselves, or sell to market; such items as pig feet, pig intestines, pig ears, pig head, chicken gizzards, chicken feet, etc. The term 'soul food' came from the fact; the slaves were given the worse food to eat. Yet they learned to cook with love and care.

Most Africans brought to the Islands of the West Indies, and the America's were taken from the West Coast of Africa. It's a natural element of a peoples culture, that they're accustomed to eat certain foods. These food diets and nutrition habits become a part of their DNA, and genetic history. When Africans were introduced to this way of life the European plantation owners forced upon them, they learned new foods to eat. Foods that today are the main cause of health ailments facing

34

African Americans, like diabetes and high blood pressure.

One's physical health in many ways, will determine their ability to earn a living.

It's no secret that medical treatment and health insurance is costly. As well as it's no secret that being not able to work for a period of time, due to illness, or an injury lessons one's ability to earn. One has to be mobile, and physically able to earn. There are them instances where a person may have a physical handicap, and still earn because their job duties, may not involve heavy lifting, standing, walking for long periods of time, or other strenuous activities. For most people, if they get injured on the job, or become ill, they'll no longer be able to work, or run their business. Exercise, is a proven method to lesson ones capacity to injury. The more fit one is, the more able one is to withstand injury, colds, other ailments, etc.

Many love money, and their physical possessions. Yet have little love for Self.

It's amazing and confusing at the same time that people will take care of their vehicle, home, jewelry and other possessions with such care, as to ensure use for a long time. When it comes to Self they act like it really doesn't matter. "We're all going to die anyway." It's a saying that I've come to believe many people hold dear too, and it's the cause for their reckless behavior, neglect of Self, and also their suffering.

Health is wealth, and the very start of ones possibilities of all manifestations to come.

VEGETARIAN

The different types of Vegetarians

Flexitarian- They eat meat occasionally, but mostly consume a plant based diet.

Pescetarian- These individuals don't consume, red meat, white meat, or fowl. Their flesh diet only consists of fish and seafood.

Pollotarian- They don't consume red meat, fish, or seafood. Their flesh diet consists of poultry and foul only.

Lacto-ovo Vegetarian- They're the most common type of vegetarians. They don't consume red meat, white meat, fish or foul. But do consume dairy products, and egg products.

Ovo Vegetarian- They only consume egg products.

Lacto Vegetarian- They only consume cheese, milk, yogurt, and retain from eating red or white meat, fish, fowl or eggs.

Vegan- They don't consume any meat products, or byproducts. Vegans don't utilize any meat products, or byproducts, in their hair care, skin care, and typically stay away from silk, leather, and wool clothing.

Who said you can't get the proteins the body needs without consuming meat

It's known that meat, and eggs are great ways to obtain protein. Both also are sources of saturated fats, and cholesterol, which can be very unhealthy.

Protein consumption is very important, as it breaks down and forms into amino acids. Amino acids promote cell growth and repair. Proteins also take longer to digest than carbohydrates. This causes you to feel fuller, and is great for anyone dieting, or exercising.

There are several food sources; one can obtain protein from besides meat, or meat byproducts. Below is a list.

Nuts, and nut butters, such as almond butter contain more than enough protein. Quinoa, cashews, spinach, oatmeal, almonds, lentil, black beans, kidney beans, pinto beans, lima beans, peas, broccoli, legumes and soy products, peanuts, brown rice, wild rice. Wheat bread is also a good source of protein. Yet bread is basically a new invention, so most vegans, don't consume any. Also, the Honorable Elijah Muhammad and Dr. Sebi do mention not to eat peanuts, and some of the other foods mentioned above.

"Honestly it took my body about ten months to adjust to not eating any beef, or chicken. I probably dropped about ten pounds within the first 40-60 days, and I was a bit weakened the first week or so by the adjustment. But I didn't notice that my appetite diminished quite a bit, and I found myself drinking more water, and being satisfied, instead of always craving food.

I was incarcerated at the time, and seventeen years old. So because, of my age my body was still going through changes. Yet by the time the first ten months came around I saw adjustments in strength, and even weight. At the time I was only about 150lbs, but I was benching 225lbs or so on the flat bench, and like 205lbs on the incline bench. My push-up, pull-up, and dip (around the world) routine was sets of 10 pull-ups, 10 dips, and I believe 20 push-ups, each go around. I would do these on my non weight days for the whole recreation period, and after lifting weights until the recreation period ended. So with personal experience I refute the belief that in order to lift weights, sports train, or be extremely active, one has to consume meat. Within four years of being a vegetarian my body weight shot up to about 175lbs, with a height of 5ft 7in. So it was basically all muscle."

VEGAN

The definition of a Vegan

Merriam dictionary Full Definition of vegan.

A strict vegetarian who consumes no animal food or dairy products; also: one who abstains from using animal products (as leather.)

The benefits of becoming a Vegan

The vegan lifestyle, is more about a philosophy about life than diet. A vegan understands that humans are mammals, and therefore, doesn't eat anything of animal origin. Nor do they utilize products of animal origin.

Today animals are injected with drugs, so they can produce at a quicker rate, which presents problems for the animal, and also produces genetically modified offspring. So, by being vegan one is supporting the right to life for all animals, mammals, etc.

Veganism, also helps the environment, and planet. The farming of animals, takes up a lot of land, and resources. The water, land, and other necessities to farm animals, could be used to feed and care for humans.

There are plenty of diseases, which are linked to animal consumption. Such as cancer, diabetes, rheumatoid arthritis, hypertension, heart disease, etc. Whole grains, vegetables, and legumes contain no cholesterol and are low in fat, especially saturated fats. There's no argument necessary when one speaks of diseases linked to animal consumption, and the lack thereof in regards to a non-meat diet. There's so much research and proof of certain diseases being the result of consuming certain types of meat. For instance, colon cancer is the result of meat not being fully digested and turning into toxic waste within the colon (large intestine.)

"Most of the people I've come across who are vegan always say it's better to start off as a vegetarian and gradually grow into becoming a vegan. At this time, I'm presently four months into the vegan move. But every now and then I find myself slipping, and eating pizza, or eggplant parmesan, eggs, and pancakes. But I've almost basically erased cakes and candy out of my diet by replacing them with nuts and fruit. I'm sure it will probably take me about another three months to get rid of the desire for cheese, and just move on with completely accomplishing a non-meat byproduct diet. I will get there, because I honestly believe in the vegan lifestyle. Hopefully, you'll follow the path too. Flesh is flesh, and I don't see eating the flesh of animals on four feet, two feet, or seafood as being any different than consuming another human."

FRUIT &

VEGETABLE CALORIES

Calories in Common Fruits & Vegetables

Food	Size	Calories
Apple	1 small (4 oz.)	80
Banana	1 medium (6 oz.)	101
Grape	each	2
Mango	1 (8 oz.)	135
Orange	1 (4 oz.)	71
Pear	1 (5 oz.)	100
Peach	1 (6 oz.)	38
Pineapple	1 cup	80
Strawberry	1 cup	53
Watermelon	1 cup	45
Asparagus	1 cup, boiled	36
Bean curd	4 oz.	81
Broccoli	1 cup	40
Carrots	1 cup	45
Cucumber	each	30
Eggplant	1 cup, boiled	38
Lettuce	1 cup	7
Tomato	1 cup	29
Egg	large	79
Shrimp, cooked	2 oz.	70
Bread, regular	1 slice (1 oz.)	75

Caesar salad	1 serving (3 cups)	360
Chocolate	1 oz.	150
Corn	1 cup, cooked	140
Potato (uncooked)	1 (6 oz.)	120
Rice, cooked	1 cup	225
Yogurt, non-fat	1 cup	150
Apricot	1 medium	20
Artichoke	1 medium	20
Asparagus	6 spears	20
Avocado	1 medium	55
Bell Pepper	1 medium	30
Blackberries	1 cup	50
Blueberries	1 cup	50
Broccoli	1 cup	20
Brussels Sprouts	4 sprouts	25
Butternut Squash	½ squash	272
Cabbage	1 cup	20
Cantaloupe	1 slice	55
Celery	1 stick	5
Cherries	1 cup	270
Corn	1 cup	60
Grapefruit	1 medium	20
Grapes	1 large bunch	310
Brussels Sprouts	4 sprouts	25
Green Beans	1 cup	30

Kale	1 cup	50
Kiwi	1 medium	40
Lettuce	1 cup	5
Nectarine	1 medium	30
Onions	1 cup	30
Papaya	1 medium	80
Peach	1 medium	40
Pear	1 medium	75
Peas	1 cup	60
Pineapple	1 cup	55
Plum	1 medium	35
Potato	1 medium	125
Radishes	1 cup	19
Raspberries	1 cup	35
Spinach	1 cup	15
Sweet potato	1 medium	60
Tomato	1 medium	20
Zucchini	1 medium	30
Butternut Squash	½ squash	272
Green Beans	1 cup	30
Kale	1 cup	50

* 1 cup = ~250 milliliters, 1 table spoon = 14.2 gram

Drugs & Alcohol

Not only are you miseducated about health, as it pertains to the whole Self (spirit, mind, body.) But you're enticed, and seduced with hallucinogens. So you can become a willing slave, and participant in your own demise.

"At 15 Years old, I smoked marijuana two times, and thought it to be ridiculous, and useless to my time, and life. How could, and why would anyone want to be in a state of confusion, and out of their normal thinking capacity? Even now, decades later I can remember thinking this. My second question to myself is why would a person spend their money, and take away from their life goals? It's equivalent to carrying out a robbery against oneself. From a business standpoint, I saw it simply as supplying the demand. But the customer side of it, I could never relate to. The two times, is my only experience with any drug use, besides an occasional aspirin or tablet, for a headache, or cold. As a young man I obtained a parole violation as a result of catching a dirty urine. This was the result of me touching and handling crack/cocaine without any protective gloves. I was at the time what one would call a street pharmacist, or entrepreneur. I couldn't tell my parole officer the reason why my urine came up with the substance in it, because of obvious reasons.

My relationship with alcohol, if that's what one will call it, didn't start until I was around 26 years old. Occasionally I would have a wine cooler, or mixed alcohol drink (hard liquor with coke, orange juice, etc.) This would be maybe 8-12 times a year. A few years it may of went up to 20 times. Necessarily, a few years ago I gradually began to disassociate myself from associates who are drinkers of liquors, and I ceased consuming alcohol. Needless to say I never needed, nor do I miss it. Nor, do I judge anyone who does consume. It's their life, and their choice. I've just decided that I'm not going to anyone's home, and hang out with them while they're consuming liquor, etc."

I honestly, believe there has always been an effort to dumb down the masses thinking capacity by keeping them high on drugs, and alcohol. It's one form of population control, because many deaths are drug and alcohol related, whether directly, or indirectly. Also most crimes, are drug and alcohol related. Every decade or so a new drug is introduced to the population, through the streets. Now, the pharmaceutical industry through the drug store market have been raking in the money, as a result of pain killers, and drugs which mimic the same high as cocaine, or heroin use. Since the people are unenlightened about their true nature. There's a lack of understanding of Self. Therefore, there's obviously a lack of respect for their own life. They really don't understand that substance abuse, or use is an actual slow form of suicide, corruption of their DNA, and weakening of their genes. Whether, they realize it or not, they pass the knowledge of this behavior on to their children. Their children are predisposed to the idea of drug, or alcohol consumption, before they even encounter the substance. So there's an emotional attachment, before it's ever been used. So a commercial, talk, or sight of the substance can trigger, the want and desire to use. Alcohol companies know this. Cigarette companies know this. The health agencies, know this about cigarettes, drugs, alcohol, and even meat. Yet, if one doesn't take the time to do their own research, they will not know what everyone, is quiet about. So each generation is becoming weaker and weaker, as a result of the consumption of eating the wrong foods, and consuming drugs in its various forms, as well being downgraded mentally, to be robots in the flesh. The masses are basically trained, what to think, instead of how to think.

The Honorable Elijah Muhammad in How to Eat to Live Part 2, mentions that government officials, civic and religious leaders know that drugs, and alcohol are deadly. Yet, they don't speak out, because they themselves are victims of the disease.

Knowledge of Self is the foundation of Self, and all other knowledge. If one doesn't have the understanding that the same intelligence, which all things evolve from resides within them as well. Then they don't realize, the power they call God, Jesus, Allah, Buddha or whatever other name, exists within them. What would truly be the use of one consuming drugs or alcohol if one understood that they're killing the God within them by taking in these pollutants? One would have to recognize this as a form of suicide; a slow form of suicide.

"As I mentioned before, my experience with drugs came from being a young hustler on the streets. I smoked marijuana two times when I was fifteen years old, and I just couldn't relate. But I saw and understand the business side of it all. So the next week a few friends and I cut out of school, got on the train and headed to Brooklyn. This was 1988, and at the time they sold $3 little manila bags. So we'd purchase them, and create $5 bags. Years later I would get into the crack/cocaine business. The lifestyle brought me in contact with all types of people, Black, White, Spanish, poor, middle class, white collar, blue collar, and business owners. I am sure of one thing. Whether, its marijuana, cocaine, crack/cocaine, prescription drugs, or heroin, drug addiction is costly to one's health and finances.

In 2001 I started working as a Quality Assurance Inspector for an over the counter (otc) drug manufacturer. In the process of learning the details of regulatory guidelines concerning packaging, I decided to take a Pharmacy Technician online course. Here I learned, all the technical terms, drug laws, classification of drugs, history, etc. The most important thing I learned was the classification of drugs, which is basically based on how the drug interacts, and affects a person's nervous system. Some prescription, and drugs sold over the counter (otc) are just as dangerous, or even more dangerous than drugs sold on the street. Liquor is a drug, and it's also sold in stores. Yet, I see it as being no different than all the other drugs on the streets. I do believe in legalizing drugs, only for the reason of being able to have it regulated like liquor, cigarettes, etc. They're all still very deadly. Yet, in the long term the public will be more educated about their choices, and Self responsibility, and the people will be able to get rid of a lot of laws, which have been designed basically to create jobs within the criminal justice system, target and terrorize minority communities with a drug war. This so called drug war is really an undercover race war. Most drug sales, are victimless crimes. An adult is responsible for their own life, and the decisions they make concerning their life. If they choose to do drugs, drink alcohol, smoke cigarettes, it's actually their choice. It may be a bad choice, but it's not the government's responsibility or power to have power over how someone maintains their health. Therefore, if they choose to do drugs, the person who sold to them, didn't force it upon them. The difference between a child, teen and adult, is more mental than physical. Legalizing drugs will definitely downsize the prison population, as there will no longer be a street market, or a very small one."

According to Treatment4Addiction.com

Drug Classifications

A drug is any substance that alters the central nervous system, brain chemistry or bodily functions. There is no single definition since there are different meanings of the word "drug", with regard to medicine, government and street usage.

Dictionary.com defines a drug as *"a chemical substance used in the treatment, cure, prevention, or diagnosis of disease or used to otherwise enhance physical or mental well-being."*

Medicinal drugs may be prescribed by a doctor for a limited time frame or for use on a regular basis for chronic condition. Recreational drugs or street drugs are drugs that target the central nervous system and brain chemistry. They are used specifically to alter perception, mood and behavior. Many recreational drugs lead to abuse and dependency. OTC refers to over-the-counter drugs, which do not require a prescription to buy.

Drug Abuse and Addiction

The Diagnostic and Statistical Manual of Mental Disorders, Fourth Edition (DSM IV) lists three stages of addiction: preoccupation/anticipation, binge/intoxication and withdrawal/negative effect. These stages are marked by cravings, obsession with and preoccupation with the substance; using more of the substance than originally intended; needing more to experience the original effect, and experiencing tolerance, withdrawal symptoms, and decreased motivation for normal life activities. It also lists two distinct addiction related disorders: abuse and dependence. Additional criteria must be met to qualify for meeting the diagnosis of dependency. When one is suffering from a drug dependency, a drug intervention is usually needed to begin the recovery process.

Drug Classifications

The vast numbers of prescribed and recreational drugs fall into certain drug classifications.

Drug Classifications:

- Stimulants (amphetamines, caffeine, nicotine and cocaine)
- Depressants (opiates and opioids, alcohol, barbiturates, tranquilizers and benzodiazepines)
- Anti-Psychotics
- Anti-Depressants
- Cannabis
- Inhalants

Prescription medications are the most commonly abuse drug in the United States.

Other Highly Abused Drugs Include:

- Nicotine and tobacco
- Crack and Cocaine
- Methamphetamine
- OxyContin (a respiratory depressant)
- Cannabis
- Heroin
- Hallucinogens
- Ecstasy and Club Drugs
- Barbiturates
- Date Rape Drugs
- Steroids

Drug Info: Top Abused Drugs

According to Jon D. Johnson, PD, MBA Vol. II No. 3 June/July 1998, the most commonly abused drugs of all types are prescription drugs.

Commonly Abuse Prescription Drugs

- Hydrocodone Combinations: Vicodin, Lorcet, Lortab, etc.
- Oxycodone Derivatives: Percodan, Percocet, Tylox, Roxicet, etc.
- Codeine Combinations
- Alprazolam (Xanax)
- Diazepam (Valium)
- Methadone
- Lorazepam (Ativan)
- Propoxyphene, Propacet,Darvocet

  Temazepam (Restoril)

- Chlordiazepoxide (Librium)

Legal Drug Classifications

You may hear of drugs being referred to as classified "Schedule 4" for example. The Controlled Substances Act of 1990 set up the Legal Classifications of drugs based on their use, abuse and how safe they are considered. The following is a partial list:

Schedule 1: High Abuse, no known medical use, Lack of Safety

Schedule 2: High Abuse, some medical use, high risk of dependency

Schedule 3: Lower abuse, medical use, and moderate dependency risk

Schedule 4: Limited abuse, high medical use, limited dependency risk

Schedule 5: Minor problems

Dependency and safety risk can rise significantly when drug interaction occurs mixing substances in different classifications. Drug overdose is also possible not only though using a large quantity but when certain drugs interact that are contraindicated. It is vitally important to have drug information that includes possible drug side effects and drug interactions.

Reality!

2013 data – About 570,000 people die annually in the U.S. due to drug use. That breaks down to about 440,000 from disease related to tobacco, 85,000 due to alcohol, 20,000 due to illicit (illegal) drugs, and 20,000 due to prescription drug abuse. If you want more information, check out NIDA's site at cdc.gov

According to National Institute on Drug Abuse for Teachers website https://teens.drugabuse.gov/national-drug-alcohol-facts-week/drug-facts-chat-day-drug-abuse

If a mother or father was addicted to drugs and then had a child, would it affect the child? Would the child have medical problems, or even be addicted to the drug?

It depends on the individual situation. There are a number of reasons why the child of addicted parents might have medical problems or become addicted. For example, if a mom is addicted to opiate drugs (like heroin, morphine, or prescription painkillers like Vicodin or OxyContin) while pregnant, her baby could be born addicted to that drug and go through a period of withdrawal. Usually this can be managed medically, but it is not a pleasant experience for the newborn (or the mom).

Researchers are also looking into whether or not exposure to other drugs before birth can make you more likely to get addicted to drugs when you are older.

So far, one researcher has found that if a mother smokes cigarettes while she is pregnant, her child is more likely to use tobacco as a teenager, and to become addicted if they do use it. The child may also have a higher risk of other medical problems like asthma, and possibly behavioral problems too. For all these reasons, we recommend that pregnant women not use alcohol or drugs, including cigarettes, during pregnancy. It they having trouble stopping drug use, they should ask their doctor for help.

Two more things that can affect your risk of addiction are genetics and family environment. If your parents are addicted to drugs, you might have a higher risk for becoming addicted yourself if you start using them. So it is especially important for kids of parents who were addicted to avoid using drugs. But the good news is if you avoid drugs, you can protect yourself from ever becoming addicted!

According to (CDC) Center for Disease Control website

http://www.cdc.gov/alcohol/fact-sheets/alcohol-use.htm

Fact Sheets - Alcohol Use and Your Health

Language:

Drinking too much can harm your health. Excessive alcohol use led to approximately 88,000 deaths and 2.5 million years of potential life lost (YPLL) each year in the United States from 2006 – 2010, shortening the lives of those who died by an average of 30 years. Further, excessive drinking was responsible for 1 in 10 deaths among working-age adults aged 20-64 years. The economic costs of excessive alcohol consumption in 2010 were estimated at $249 billion, or $2.05 a drink.

What is a "drink"?

In the United States, a standard drink contains 0.6 ounces (14.0 grams or 1.2 tablespoons) of pure alcohol. Generally, this amount of pure alcohol is found in

12-ounces of beer (5% alcohol content).

8-ounces of malt liquor (7% alcohol content).

5-ounces of wine (12% alcohol content).

1.5-ounces of 80-proof (40% alcohol content) distilled spirits or liquor (e.g., gin, rum, vodka, whiskey).[4]

What is excessive drinking?

Excessive drinking includes binge drinking, heavy drinking, and any drinking by pregnant women or people younger than age 21.

Binge drinking, the most common form of excessive drinking, is defined as consuming

For women, 4 or more drinks during a single occasion.

For men, 5 or more drinks during a single occasion.

Heavy drinking is defined as consuming

For women, 8 or more drinks per week.

For men, 15 or more drinks per week.

Most people who drink excessively are not alcoholics or alcohol dependent.

What is moderate drinking?

The **Dietary Guidelines for Americans** defines moderate drinking as up to 1 drink per day for women and up to 2 drinks per day for men.[4] In addition, the **Dietary Guidelines** do not recommend that individuals who do not drink alcohol start drinking for any reason.

However, there are some people who should **not** drink any alcohol, including those who are:

Younger than age 21.

Pregnant or may be pregnant.

Driving, planning to drive, or participating in other activities requiring skill, coordination, and alertness.

Taking certain prescription or over-the-counter medications that can interact with alcohol.

Suffering from certain medical conditions.

Recovering from alcoholism or are unable to control the amount they drink.

By adhering to the **Dietary Guidelines**, you can reduce the risk of harm to yourself or others.

Short-Term Health Risks

Excessive alcohol use has immediate effects that increase the risk of many harmful health conditions. These are most often the result of binge drinking and include the following:

Injuries, such as motor vehicle crashes, falls, drownings, and burns.

Violence, including homicide, suicide, sexual assault, and intimate partner violence.

Alcohol poisoning, a medical emergency that results from high blood alcohol levels.

Risky sexual behaviors, including unprotected sex or sex with multiple partners. These behaviors can result in unintended pregnancy or sexually transmitted diseases, including HIV.

Miscarriage and stillbirth or fetal alcohol spectrum disorders (FASDs) among pregnant women.

Long-Term Health Risks

Over time, excessive alcohol use can lead to the development of chronic diseases and other serious problems including:

High blood pressure, heart disease, stroke, liver disease, and digestive problems.

Cancer of the breast, mouth, throat, esophagus, liver, and colon.

Learning and memory problems, including dementia and poor school performance.

Mental health problems, including depression and anxiety.

Social problems, including lost productivity, family problems, and unemployment.

Alcohol dependence, or alcoholism.

By not drinking too much, you can reduce the risk of these short- and long-term health risks.

EXERCISE

There's a saying that goes "What You Don't Use, You Lose."

As one ages, their bodies' mobility has a lot to do with how active they've remained throughout their life. Exercise, doesn't only mean lifting weights. It can also according to the dictionary be, bodily or mental exertion, especially for the sake of training or improvement of health: Walking is good exercise. 2. something done or performed as a means of practice or training: exercises for the piano.

"In school I was athletic. I can remember being in elementary school and being the second fastest in the district to run the 100 yard dash. This lasted all the way up to sixth grade. By the time I reached Junior High School, the gym teacher was trying to recruit me to join the wrestling team.

At the age of seventeen I would get incarcerated and from this point, I started lifting weights and doing calisthenics (push-ups, pull-ups) etc. Exercise, is definitely one form of stress reliever. During this age in my life, I had a lot of aggression, and I would go work out whenever I needed to clear my head of negative thoughts. This was on top of my normal routines. Exercise and being active has been, and will always be a part of my life."

Obesity, is a very big health issue in America. Aside from unhealthy eating habits, most people don't exercise. Everyone comes out the house, gets in their car, truck, or on their motorcycle, and goes on their way. This is so, even if their destination is only around the corner. Even in school, gym class is like a chore, instead of part of one's daily activity.

Exercising is for more than just looking good

When one exercises endomorphins are released. Endomorphins according to the dictionary are, any of a group of hormones secreted within the brain and nervous system and having a number of physiological functions. They are peptides that activate the body's opiate receptors, causing an analgesic effect.

In other words, exercise helps one feel good. This obviously helps one think more positively, and focus more. People who exercise tend to be more driven, and the get up and go type.

When ones idea about Self evolves, so does their understanding of health.

If one understands that their body is their temple, and houses their spirit. They'll also realize the importance of taking care of their physical composition, through eating healthy and exercising.

"At the time of writing this book I'm 45 years old. I weigh 158lbs, and I'm not nearly as bulky as I was 15 years ago and back. I'm healthy though, and very active. Being out and about selling my books, I'm always on foot, going here and there. I find that it's better to be on foot in some areas, because I can go store to store, and also meet people on the street as they walk. Right now my exercise routines consists of walking, riding a bicycle, push-ups, weightless squats, stretches, and stomach exercises once in a while. 3-4 times a week, I engage in the push up and weightless squat routines. My body is ripped like Bruce Lee. I believe, even more so than he. I'd be lying if I didn't say I feel good. The best part is people mistake me all the time for being at least 10 years younger than my age. Many people I know in their 40's are experiencing weight, and other health problems, as a result of their food diet, and social lifestyles (drugs, alcohol, etc.)I'm a person who believes that all circumstances are the product of cause and effect. It was obvious to me as a young person, that from watching people with drug addiction, alcohol addiction, weight problems, diabetes, and other ailments that I really wanted little to do with bad health. So I decided to be concerned in thought and action, about how I took care of myself. It just seemed like the sensible thing to do."

Moderate intensity aerobic activity, like walking is generally safe for most people. Heart attacks happen rarely when people are physically active. But there is risk when you suddenly become much more active, then you're used to. One may need to work with a personal trainer, or consult with their doctor. It's very important to know one's own mental, physical health, preparedness, strengths and weaknesses.

Chronic health conditions, such as arthritis, diabetes, or heart disease, may limit one's ability to be active. Contact your doctor and discuss what activity is best. Nevertheless, the benefits of exercise far outweigh ones risks of being injured.

Aside from maintaining a healthy diet, exercise is the next best thing for the body.

Conclusion

Health is wealth. I'll save the long explanation about the contents of the book, because I'm certain I've made the point very clear.

People of African descent in the Americas must change the way they think, eat and live in order to truly change their circumstances. They must realign their consciousness and DNA with the ancient Self, in order to be complete in spirit, mind and body, in the present.

Caucasians, and the other human families, must acknowledge that they've been deceived about Self, and the relationship between the spirit, mind and body, working as one for total health of all individuals. One cannot eat poisonous foods, drug, and drink, and expect not to affect their consciousness, DNA, and future genetic history. One cannot be treated for an ailment, and be given medication to only treat the physical symptoms. This is only a remedy, as it doesn't also deal with the metaphysical aspect of the individual. Corporate greed has tainted he political, civic and spiritual leaders to the point, where they acknowledge that western society is living in a culture of Self destruction. Yet, they will not speak up because, of their own weaknesses, and the fact that they themselves profit financially. The food and pharmaceutical industry are powerful within the political arena, and also Wall Street.

72